VEGAN

The Ultimate Beginner's Guide To The Vegan Diet

By Nicholas Welby

Copyright © 2017 Nicholas Welby

All rights reserved.

This book or any portion thereof may not be reproduced or used in any manner whatsoever without the express written permission of the publisher except for the use of brief quotations in a book review.

This book is not intended as a substitute for the medical advice of physicians. The reader should regularly consult a physician in matters relating to his/her health and particularly with respect to any symptoms that may require diagnosis or medical attention.

Printed in the United States of America

Table of Contents

Introduction 5
Chapter 1: What Is Veganism, and Where Did It Come From? 7
Chapter 2: Health Benefits of a Vegan Diet 12
Chapter 3: Frequently Asked Questions About Veganism 16
Chapter 4: Myths About the Vegan Diet 18
Chapter 5: Rules Vegans Live By – and Which Foods to Avoid 21
Chapter 6: Grocery Store Essentials for a Vegan Diet 25
Chapter 7: Seven-Day Meal Plan for Good Vegan Health 29
Chapter 8: Eating Out 34
Chapter 9: Tips and Tricks to Help You Stay on a Vegan Diet 41
Conclusion 45

Introduction

The vegan lifestyle is not as new as many people think – vegans have been choosing to avoid animal products for health and ethical reasons for hundreds of years. So why are plant-based diets currently receiving more attention than ever before?

There can seem to be thousands of bloggers and vloggers promoting the health benefits of a vegan lifestyle online, and these are proving particularly popular with younger people. Vegan recipe books and specialist ingredients are easier to come by than ever before. Documentaries and films are also being made to attempt to persuade us that meat and dairy are not just bad for people, but also the planet. Overall, there has never been so much information available about the many and varied reasons to go vegan.

All the noise around veganism can, however, make the idea of actually trying a vegan diet seem rather overwhelming. Do you have to be an eco-warrior to go vegan? Will it be possible to eat out? Will everyone you know think you've gone crazy? Is veganism just a dangerous trend which can lead to disordered eating? Amongst all the vegan celebrities, advertisements for nutritional supplements, specialist products, and media hypes, it can be very hard to get a sense of what it is actually like to be a vegan.

This guide aims to set out the facts about veganism and to dispel a few myths so that you can weigh up the information available and make the right lifestyle choice for you and your circumstances. If you want to inform yourself about a plant-based, vegan diet, then read on.

CHAPTER 1

What Is Veganism, and Where Did It Come From?

From health food shops to social media, it seems that meat- and dairy-free options are now more easily available than ever before. There is a greater awareness of lactose intolerance, and a better understanding of the importance of whole foods for a healthy, well-rounded diet. But why would someone choose to go completely vegan? Veganism seems to be the latest trend at the moment, and many people have an opinion on whether this diet is beneficial or overly restrictive. Looking at the roots of veganism shows that it is not as unified as other types of diets – there is no one book which is the vegan 'bible'. For as long as veganism has existed, there have been different reasons for people for cut out animal products, and many sub-sets of veganism itself.

So where did veganism begin? Well, believe it or not, the vegan diet did not begin with YouTube bloggers or wholefood shoppers! Many philosophers and religious devotees around the world have chosen to follow a plant-based diet throughout recorded history. This has sometimes been due to particular beliefs about animals or caring for the environment, or simply because this type of natural food was felt to be beneficial to deep thought and prayer. Some Rastafarians, Jains, and other religious practitioners still choose a vegan diet for spiritual reasons.

Only a minority of new vegans these days may have turned to a plant-based diet for religious reasons. But with diseases and disorders on the rise and increasing concerns about food production methods, many people are asking serious questions about what they put in their bodies. It is this interest in good health and nutrition that accounts for the largest part of the rise in veganism.

Perhaps one of the main reasons that people are more interested in healthful living than ever before is, paradoxically, that we are all living longer and have become accustomed to expecting medical science to solve our health problems.

However, as we are now less likely to die from the sort of environmental factors which shorted our grandparent's lives, such as smoking, exhausting manual labor, and preventable diseases, we are now facing different illnesses and issues. Sometimes these illnesses are a natural part of life, but sometimes they are avoidable, or even caused by modern society. The excessive consumption of fatty and sugary foods, use of toxic substances in commercial food production, lack of exercise and stress associated with today's patterns of living and working are all connected to contemporary killers such as cancer, heart disease, obesity, and depression.

Meanwhile, medicine is advancing but also becoming expensive. We expect to live longer, but don't want to spend our retirement in discomfort or being a burden to others. Little wonder then that we are increasingly looking to the cause rather than treatment of social and medical problems – diet.

The actual term 'vegan' didn't emerge until the founding of the Vegan Society and its newsletter in the UK in 1944. An American Vegan Society followed a few years after, and the idea of veganism as a distinct grouping of beliefs and practices has been evolving ever since.

It is important to bear in mind that, for as long as veganism has existed, there have been different reasons for avoiding animal products, which can affect what is meant by the term 'vegan'. The most frequently seen approaches to veganism can probably be categorized as follows:

1. Dietary Veganism

Dietary vegans simply avoid all animal products and by-products in their diet, including meat but also dairy and eggs. They are also likely to avoid animal by-products such as honey, beeswax, animal-based colorants and flavors, and so on. Sometimes the term 'plant-based' is used to show that someone takes a vegan approach to their diet, but is not so engaged in the more political aspects of veganism. This approach to a vegan diet is often chosen primarily for reasons of health and nutrition.

2. Ethical Veganism

A broader view of veganism is taken by many followers of this diet, whereby animal products and exploitation are avoided in all possible areas of life. Ethical vegans may avoid wearing leather or wool, buying makeup and skin products which involve animal-based ingredients or testing. It may also affect how they approach other lifestyle choices such as visiting a zoo or owning a pet.

This approach to veganism can seem isolating, as it involves such a different approach to shopping and leisure time, as well as food. However, with the increasing popularity of veganism and campaigns around animal rights, there is perhaps more of a sense of community for ethical and political vegans than ever before. Some towns and cities have several vegan cafes and businesses, and there are many online communities too. Joining a forum or visiting a local vegetarian or vegan café might help you see what exists in your area.

3. Raw Veganism

Raw veganism is exactly what it sounds like because raw vegans eat only (or mostly) raw plant foods. This is definitely a less popular approach to veganism, but more and more people have been trying it over the last few years. One reason for this is no doubt the popularity of the paleo diet, which, while it is certainly not necessarily vegan, does promote the consumption of natural, unprocessed foods. Raw foods are seen to be closer to what nature would have intended for humans, and therefore gentler on our digestive systems and less likely to cause diseases such as cancer.

Another reason that raw veganism is becoming more visible is that it is now much easier to obtain fresh fruits and vegetables all year round in many parts of the world, making raw food more accessible in climates where fresh goods would otherwise be seasonal only. Raw vegans will definitely need to supplement their diet with other types of food and nutritional additives in order to remain healthy.

4. Fruitarianism and Other More Restrictive Variants of Veganism

There are some dietary practices which appear to overlap with veganism but are in fact far more restrictive. Fruitarians, for example, eat a diet of which a very large proportion is fresh fruit, but they will often also include nuts, seeds, powders, and other supplements. Fruitarianism is not appropriate for children or teenagers, and anyone considering these more unusual diets for more than a short-term detox would benefit from seeking nutritional advice.

So veganism seems to have only a few simple rules, and yet it is complicated by the various reasons people have for adopting this way of eating. That isn't a bad thing, though – it shows that even with an apparently restrictive dietary approach such as veganism, there is a lot of room for all types of people. Whatever your lifestyle, beliefs, or background, there is probably a way to be vegan which can promote good health for you.

In order to navigate questions such as whether you will eat honey or want to experiment with raw smoothies, ask yourself: what is it about veganism that appeals to you? Do you like to make ethical decisions in life? Do you feel strongly about animal rights? Are you a bodybuilder looking for a healthier relationship with protein? Do you love fruits and vegetables and want to incorporate them more into your diet? Are there particular health problems which you are hoping to address or avoid? Veganism has answers to all those questions and a whole lot more too!

CHAPTER 2

Health Benefits of a Vegan Diet

Veganism is increasing in popularity, but it is a very different way of eating to the standard Western diet. It is therefore important to do research and prepare yourself if you are considering a plant-based approach to food so that you can decide whether it's for you, how to make the change, and what potential problems you ought to be aware of.

Whether or not you have an interest in the ethical aspects of veganism, or are primarily motivated by the nutritional benefits, there is no doubt that this diet has proven health-promoting qualities. The most well-publicized benefit of eating a plant-based diet is the reduction in the chances of developing major health problems, which can include:

- Heart disease
- Diabetes
- Inflammatory and digestive disorders
- Degenerative and neurological problems
- Some types of cancer

A vegan diet can also help manage ongoing health conditions, such as:

- Eczema and other skin disorders
- Irritable bowel syndrome and leaky gut
- Constipation
- High cholesterol
- Sluggishness and low energy
- Depression and anxiety

There are many reasons why a vegan diet can promote good health in such a wide variety of ways, but they can be summarized in the following ways:

More Fruits and Vegetables Means More Vitamins for Your Body

A *balanced* vegan diet generally includes more vitamins and minerals from all the fresh fruits and vegetables you probably eat more of as a vegan, compared to someone eating a typical modern diet. It is thought that before industrialization and large-scale agriculture were developed, berries and other wild vegetable foods made up the largest part of our diet. Our teeth are designed for cutting and chewing through nuts, fruits, and greens, rather than the flesh of animals. It is therefore unsurprising that eating in this way seems to suit the human body.

Fresh fruits contain a lot of vitamin C, which can help keep minor infections at bay and support you to feel well in general. Many fruits also contain antioxidants, which are thought to fight the free radical associated with cancer and the development of pre-cancerous cells. These vitamins also work wonders for how you feel on the outside – vitamins and antioxidants are important for the health of your skin. Consuming lots of fresh fruit and choosing skin products which use plant-based ingredients can help prevent acne, and slow down the breakdown of collagen and elastin in the skin. So eating vegan could help you look younger while living longer!

Some Animal Products Are Known Carcinogens

It has been shown that the consumption of many animal-based food products correlates with higher rates of particular diseases. The World Health Organization has stated that many processed meats, including smoked bacon, sausages, and other similar products, are a cause of cancer. Even if you aren't sure about making a transition to a fully vegan diet, you should definitely consider cutting out processed meats and animal products which have been produced in chemical-laden environments.

Meat, Dairy, and Eggs Are Strongly Connected to Higher Levels of Cholesterol

Because many animal products are sources of highly saturated fats, they contribute to the build-up of cholesterol in the body. Cholesterol makes it harder for oxygen to get around the body, and puts a strain on the heart as it tries to pump blood through clogged veins and arteries. It can therefore lead to heart disease and heart attack, as well as stroke. Cholesterol is a silent killer because there are few symptoms of high cholesterol itself, but the complications it leads to are serious or fatal. Taking dietary measures to reduce your levels of cholesterol is therefore one of the biggest steps you can take towards a longer, healthier life. And while there are certainly vegan sources of cholesterol, cutting out meat and dairy is a simple and easy way to avoid some of the biggest culprits for high rates of heart disease.

Diabetes and Associated Risks

There is increasing evidence that eating a vegan diet is likely to promote the ability of the body to deal with insulin. With rates of type 2 diabetes on the rise in many parts of the world, any dietary change which can help avoid diabetes and its serious complications is worthy of consideration.

Whilst diabetes is a manageable condition, its long-term effects can seriously affect your quality of life and even become life-threatening. Common problems associated with diabetes range from tingling in the extremities and digestive problems, to blindness, stroke, nerve damage and ulcers, kidney disease, and heart attack. Sexual function and fertility can also be affected, so while it might not be immediately life-threatening, diabetes is certainly a condition to be taken seriously and managed as well as possible.

Alkalinity and Inflammation

Why is it that a vegan diet seems to be so healthful in general? Well, many people believe it is because a plant-based diet promotes alkalinity, while meat- and dairy-based diets are more heavily acidic. That acidity can irritate the digestive tract and cause inflammation in cells, which is thought to make them more vulnerable to some types of cancer, particularly in the colon.

Digestive problems don't just affect the digestive function itself, but also many other aspects of good health. If food moves through the digestive tract too quickly, the body doesn't have time to absorb all the nutrients it needs. If the delicate balance of gut bacteria and pH levels is not quite right, the enzymes which allow energy and nutrients to be absorbed cannot function efficiently. Of course, the results can be wide-ranging, because all parts of the body require good nutrition in order to work to their full potential and fight off disease.

The 'Feel-Good' Factor

Some proponents of veganism suggest it also has a spiritual or karmic aspect. They believe that, by not eating products which are involved in animal killing or exploitation, negative energy and connotations of death or depression are kept out of the system. There is no reliable research in this area, and whether or not it is a relevant aspect of veganism is a subjective matter for the individual.

CHAPTER 3

Frequently Asked Questions About Veganism

As veganism becomes more widespread, it is easier to identify the main queries and concerns people may have about this approach to food. Here is a selection of the most common queries people raise when they are considering going vegan:

Q: Is a vegan diet hard to follow?

A: There is no denying that a vegan diet is quite different to the average Western diet, and that can make it a bit of a shock – both to your digestive system and your lifestyle. Many people get around this by planning a transition period, during which they gradually remove animal-based products from their diet. For example, you might start by going vegetarian for a few weeks or months, before cutting out dairy products. But if you are committed and passionate, there are no real obstacles to changing to a vegan diet whenever you want.

Q: There aren't any specialist vegan shops near me, so how can I go vegan?

A: If this is the only thing stopping you from trying a vegan diet, why not check out online vegan shops? There are many mail-order and virtual wholefood supply services which you can use to get hold of any ingredients you can't find locally. And while specialist vegan foods can be convenient, they really aren't necessary. A good vegan diet, like any other healthy approach to eating, should include plenty of wholefoods, so the more meals you can prepare yourself, the better!

Q: Are there groups of people who shouldn't go vegan?

A: This is a good question because it is true that each person is different. But there are very few people indeed who cannot live healthily on a vegan diet. While there will always be exceptions to every rule, there are groups who will need to focus on particular nutritional requirements when they're on a plant-based diet, such as women of child-bearing age (who need higher rates of iron to avoid anemia), pregnant and breastfeeding women, babies, and toddlers. The only people for whom a vegan diet simply is not possible are those who have to avoid large food groups due to other pre-existing medical conditions or major allergies. This is not because a vegan diet would be 'bad' for this group of people, but simply because it may be difficult for all nutritional requirements to be met when a diet is already restricted.

Q: Is it possible for a fussy eater, or someone who doesn't much like vegetables, to go vegan?

This is perhaps the most common reason that people put off going vegan. It can be very hard to imagine enjoying a diet if it's full of food you don't usually eat. However, there are two good responses commonly given to this. One is that whatever currently features in your diet to the exclusion of vegetables, whether that's meat or junk food or bread, should be something which you aim to reduce or give up for your health. You may not like the idea of giving it up, but if veganism appeals to you, then you will see why it could be worthwhile.

The other response is that we are very adaptable, and foods which currently seem unexciting should, once you have adapted to them, become familiar. You will learn your favorite ways to prepare them, and which other foods to serve them with so that you can enjoy your meal. Veganism is often viewed as a diet of self-limitation, but in fact, it is simply a matter of adaptation.

CHAPTER 4

Myths About the Vegan Diet

There are many myths about the vegan diet, and many of them come from the fact that it is such a different way of eating to the average Western diet. If you can educate yourself about some common misconceptions before becoming vegan, you will be able to make your decisions – and reassure any relatives and co-workers who may have concerns.

"It's hard to get enough protein if you don't eat meat!"

Perhaps the most frequently expressed worry is that it is difficult to get enough protein on a vegan diet. However, this myth is based on the prevalence of meat eating in most parts of the world. Did you know that animals don't actually make protein, but take it in from plants lower down the food chain? A vegan diet allows you to skip the 'middle man' and access protein sources directly.

It is true that vegans should ensure that their diet includes a range of sources of protein, such as beans, legumes, and nuts, and the many other options which can be combined in a number of tasty ways. It is also true that many omnivores eat more protein than they really need, and that excess protein doesn't benefit the body at all. Only athletes, bodybuilders, and other people who put their bodies through unusual amounts of exertion on a daily basis need to worry about protein.

"Vegans are more likely to suffer broken bones when they get older!"

Another myth vegans often hear is that they might not receive enough calcium, and will end up suffering from arthritis or osteoporosis. We are used to thinking that milk, cheese, and other dairy products are what 'makes' bones, but the processes involved in bone health can be supported in many ways. After all, the human digestive system was not designed around cow's milk! Vegan sources of calcium include soy milk (which is often fortified with calcium and other nutrients), chia seeds, kale, and many other plant-based products.

Pregnant and breastfeeding women may need to be extra vigilant about their nutrition, however. A growing baby will take whatever nutrients it needs from its mother so, if the mother's diet does not adequately provide for both, the nutrients will be taken from her own stores. It is perfectly possible to be vegan throughout this time – after all, many parts of the world have high rates of lactose intolerance and women there manage this period without nutritional problems – but extra research and planning should be undertaken for those new to this way of eating.

"Vegans have strange bowel habits and tend to be gassy!"

They might be too polite to say it, but many people are curious about the impact of a vegan diet on 'regularity'! However, the regularity of bowel movements should not be a concern for those on a vegan diet. Most medical experts state that the normal rate is very varied – some people go a few times a day, other people every few days.

Vegans often find that they are much less prone to the discomfort and bloating associated with constipation, because a plant-based diet is naturally very high in fiber. Fiber is the binding substance which helps food move through in a way which supports optimal absorption of nutrients. A vegan diet is therefore ideal for people who suffer from digestive discomfort or irregular bowels.

As for gassiness, well, it's not a real health concern, but some people may find it socially unacceptable! Some types of food may cause gas for different people, but there are natural ways to deal with that if need be. Taking digestive enzymes, or drinking a calming tea such as ginger or fennel, will all aid good digestion and help with any gas issues.

"If you are vegan, you probably have an eating disorder!"

If you are considering a vegan diet, it is likely to be for a combination of reasons related to health, nutrition, and perhaps the environment too. It might therefore come as a surprise to find that some people can be quite critical of veganism for a wide range of reasons. Some people seem to think that because a vegan diet excludes the intake of entire types of food, it suggests an individual has an unhealthy relationship with food. This is really the result of ignorance – we are not taught through schools or mainstream media that our nutritional requirements can be met through a plant-based diet, so many people react with aversion or concern. If your friends or family seem concerned, just direct them towards informative material, such as this guide, and get on with living your life so that you become an example of a happy, healthy vegan. If you should meet anyone who is truly judgmental or rude, you may have to find ways to distance yourself from their opinion.

CHAPTER 5

Rules Vegans Live By – and Which Foods to Avoid

The rules of veganism appear straightforward compared to many other diets and detoxes. Surely, it's simple – just don't eat anything which comes from an animal! But the thing about veganism is, it's as much about what you *should* eat as what you shouldn't eat. The increasing availability of vegan convenience foods is great for those who need them, but it makes it easy to miss out on essential nutrients if you aren't mindful in your choices. Plant-based ingredients such as palm oil are also very often used in low-cost junk foods – which can be great from time to time, but those Oreos will not contribute to a healthy lifestyle!

So with a vegan diet, the rules to live by are not so much *don'ts* as *do's* – remembering the food groups and nutrients which need to be part of a balanced diet. Here is a list of the most important nutrients which your body needs, and the food groups you can eat to ensure a balanced diet.

Important Vegan Nutrients
Protein

Protein is a key building block of the human body, and is also used to help it repair and defend itself against injury and disease. Protein can be found in:

- Tofu
- Lentils
- Kidney beans
- Peas
- Broccoli
- Soy milk and desserts
- Nuts and seeds

Iron

Iron deficiency is common in many diets, but easy to avoid if you know which vegan foods are rich in iron. The iron in food is more easily absorbed – or 'bioavailable' – when the body also has a good supply of vitamin C. It is therefore a good idea to also eat citrus fruits or drink some orange juice after a meal rich in iron. Great vegan sources of iron include:

- Fortified breakfast cereals
- Kale
- Dried fruits, especially apricots and raisins
- Lentils and chickpeas
- Many types of seed
- Cashew nuts

Vitamin D and B12

Vitamin D is important for bone health, and B12 keeps your nervous system healthy and stops you from feeling tired. While the body can produce vitamin D from exposure to the sun, you may wish to use a supplement if you don't live in a sunny climate for at least part of the year. B12 is another nutrient for which there is no known natural source for vegans. You should therefore either include plenty of fortified foods such as bread and cereal in your diet, or look for a good vegan-friendly supplement.

Junk Food and the Vegan Diet

It is surprising how many convenience and junk foods are meat- and dairy-free. This is partly because more people are limiting their intake of animal products, but also because for many types of cheap junk food, plant-based oils make production cheaper. These foods often include cookies, potato chips, crackers, and fries. Whilst it is fine to have these things in moderation as part of any balanced diet, those considering a vegan diet must be aware that just because an ingredient is plant-based, it does not automatically mean that the product is healthy.

In fact, some of the most widely used ingredients in foods associated with obesity and heart disease are plant-based. Here is a list of a few ingredients which vegans should be aware of when incorporating processed foods into their diet:

Palm Oil

Palm oil is produced in many parts of the world and widely used as a fat throughout the commercial food industry because of its low cost and stability. However, this stability is due to the fact that palm oil is very high in saturated fats. Palm oil also contains palmitic acid and studies suggest that, in combination with the high levels of fat, that makes palm oil a contributing factor in high cholesterol and associated heart diseases.

There are also environmental concerns about the production of palm oil, because of the way natural forests and other plants have been cleared in order to grow the number of palm trees required by the food industry. This factor is of concern to some ethical vegans.

Corn Syrup

Corn syrup is a commercial sweetener and stabilizer used by commercial producers in many popular foods, but particularly products where sugar would generally be used. Common uses for corn syrup are candy, pancake syrup, desserts, and sauces. These are of course all foods which, if consumed to excess, will lead to obesity and all the complications associated with excessive weight gain.

However, there is one type of corn syrup which is particularly important to avoid. High-fructose corn syrup is a form of corn syrup which has undergone further chemical processes in order to produce a much sweeter taste. High-fructose corn syrup is therefore used in the products where people most expect a sugary taste – cans of soda and fizzy soft drinks. Anyone trying to live a healthy lifestyle should try to cut out, or at least restrict, their intake of soda, as a can of soda contains the equivalent of up to 15 teaspoons of sugar. High-fructose corn syrup is also produced in chemical-laden environments. The process involves heavy metals like mercury, which are very toxic for humans.

If you do decide to go vegan and find yourself craving sugary or junk foods, ask yourself whether you need to address any other deficiencies in your diet or lifestyle. Maybe you aren't getting enough sleep or need to check your B12 intake. Make any changes needed to ensure you don't rely on junk foods to get through the day!

Other Suspicious Ingredients

Vegans often regard themselves as taking a more conscious approach to diet. That means that researching and choosing healthy and non-exploitative foods is more fundamental than choosing one food group over another, or being specific about portion control. If you are drawn to this conscious consumer approach, you will also want to be vigilant about other ingredients which can be hidden inside foods targeted at vegans.

Just because something is labelled 'natural' or 'organic', it doesn't mean you can stop being careful. Some countries have quite loose legal definitions of these terms, and you will still need to read the ingredients list if you want to be sure you aren't putting something unhealthy into your body. Vegans will often choose to try and avoid genetically modified produce, foods containing MSG, and other ingredients which are known to be bad for the environment and ourselves.

CHAPTER 6

Grocery Store Essentials for a Vegan Diet

If you're new to eating vegan, you will also be new to shopping vegan. Simply trying to switch out anything you usually buy for plant-based alternatives means you'd miss out on the nutritional benefits of many wholefoods. It would also be expensive, and probably not very tasty! So here are some suggestions for store cupboard essentials which many vegans like to keep around. You can use these to put together a wide range of fantastic meals for you, your family, and your friends.

Pulses

Pulses and legumes are vital sources of protein on a vegan diet. Many people associate these foods with plain dahl and soups, but there are so many types that it is worth exploring all the flavors and textures available. Besides the traditional Eastern cuisine, you can also try stirring pulses into stews, pasta dishes, and salads to make those more substantial. Why not try:

- Lentils: Orange, green, speckled, and many other varieties too!
- Chana Dhal makes an economical side dish or lunch with your favorite spices added
- Dried peas make a good soup when fresh peas aren't available
- Kidney beans are the ideal alternative to beef in a chili
- Chickpeas stirred in lemon juice, olive oil, and coriander are wonderful in a salad. Or blend it up for some fresh hummus!
- Add some butter beans to a soup or casserole for a lovely creamy texture

Grains

Grains are an important source of carbohydrates, fiber, and protein. Choose wholegrain options such as brown rice where you can, as those won't have had their naturally occurring nutrients removed with excessive processing.

- Rice is a staple food around the world for good reason – it is nourishing and adaptable. From curries to risottos and salads, make sure to keep a few varieties on hand. Fragrant rice such as jasmine can be lovely to

balance a curry, while specialist rice for sushi and risotto will come in useful too.
- Quinoa – anytime you are cooking up some grains, consider adding a little quinoa to the mix. It will bring a nice nutty flavor and is a complete source of protein.
- Less common grains such as bulgur wheat, millet, and linseed are all fantastic sources of minerals that add a lot of texture and color to everything from pastry flour to crumble toppings. You will probably need to visit a specialist shop to find a good range.

Nuts, Seeds, and Dried Fruits

Dried foods are often associated with the stereotypical 'hippy', so many people assume that they must be tasteless and boring. This couldn't be further from the truth! Besides being a tasty snack and addition to meals, these foods are sources of many nutrients, including selenium, iron, calcium, and protein. It can be worth buying your favorites in bulk and making up a custom trail mix – not only is it easy on the budget, but it means you can mix up something you know your whole family will enjoy. You can also tailor it to your specific nutritional needs by including particular seeds or fortified cereal.

Here are suggestions for ingredients to stock up on:
- Chia, pumpkin, and sunflower seeds
- Brazil and cashew nuts for snacking
- Peanuts – but be sure to choose an unsalted version
- Raisins, apricots, dried figs, prunes, cherries, goji berries, cranberries, and dates
- Cereal hoops or flakes fortified with B12 and iron – but try to avoid varieties which have lots of added sugar

Egg Substitutes

New vegans often find it difficult to go without eggs not just because they are a source of protein, but because they have a variety of culinary uses. Luckily, there are many vegan substitutes for egg, some of which are available in ready-made form at specialist shops. These can be very convenient and easy to use, especially for cake recipes. But they can be less cost-effective and harder to obtain than home-made alternatives.

There is no one perfect substitute for eggs, because they are used in so many different ways. Some types of recipe will work best with a fruit-based substitute, whilst other require something with lighter or raising properties. So there can be a bit of a learning curve to replacing eggs, but it is certainly possible to make cakes, batter, sauces, and anything else you can think of on a vegan diet.

Here is a list of egg substitutes which can be sourced or made at home, and adapted to your own recipe. Each quantity is equal to one egg, but some experimentation may be helpful to find the best fit for a particular recipe.

1. For recipes which use egg to 'bind' ingredients together such as pancakes, sauces, and 'meat' balls:
   - 1 tablespoon ground flax (linseed) blended with 3 tablespoons of water
   - 1 tablespoon soy protein powder stirred into 3 tablespoons of water
   - Half a mashed banana
   - ¼ cup of pureed apple or unsweetened apple sauce
   - 3 tablespoons peanut butter
2. For recipes which use egg to 'set', such as puddings and cheesecakes:
   - 1 tablespoon agar agar and 1 tablespoon water
   - 1 tablespoon chia seeds mixed into 1/3 cup of water and left to sit for fifteen minutes
3. For recipes which use egg to 'raise' such as cupcakes:
   - 1 tablespoon vinegar (white vinegar or apple cider vinegar are fine) and 1 tablespoon baking soda

Experimenting with new ingredients is one of the most exciting aspects of going vegan, so don't let the range of possibilities intimidate you! You will come to learn which ingredients you rely on, and the best places to find them in your area.

CHAPTER 7

Seven-Day Meal Plan for Good Vegan Health

Unlike other diets, veganism doesn't specify a certain number of calories, or that you should weigh your foods, or only eat certain food groups at certain times. The 'rules' are much simpler, but it can involve such a big change from our usual eating habits that many people struggle to imagine what vegans actually eat! So below is an example meal plan for someone on a vegan diet. It does not focus on any particular goal such as weight loss or muscle building, but it can easily be adapted to individual needs.

Monday
- Breakfast: Start your week off with an energy-boosting smoothie made from fruits which are high in Vitamin C and a handful of kale. If you are heading to the gym, you could add your favorite protein powder. If you're prone to mid-morning snacking, pack a couple of slices of wholegrain bread spread with a soy-based cream cheese alternative and a few cherry tomatoes.
- Lunch: Pitta breads filled with hummus, lettuce, and cucumber. Add a couple of oatcakes to see you through until your evening meal.
- Dinner: Baked sweet potatoes with a kidney bean chili and side salad. Follow up with a fresh fruit salad for balance.

Tuesday
- Breakfast: Two slices of toast spread with mashed avocado. Sprinkle on some salt, pepper, lemon juice, and sesame and chia seeds for a nutrient hit.
- Lunch: Pack yourself a healthy version of the classic peanut butter and jelly sandwich, using nutrient-dense ingredients such as wholegrain bread, sunflower oil spread, pure ground peanut butter without the added sugar, and maybe some homemade jam if you have it!
- Dinner: Stir-fry tonight – toss some sliced tofu in corn flour and soy sauce before frying it up with your favorite Chinese veggies and some rice noodles. While that's cooking, stuff cored baking apples with

raisins and toss them into the oven to bake for an hour. Serve with a drizzle of maple syrup, and you won't go hungry anytime soon!

Wednesday
- Breakfast: If you find you start to flag around the middle of the week, get out those porridge oats. Slowly cook them up in almond milk, and add some chopped dried apricots and a spoonful of vegan chocolate spread to set you up for the day.
- Lunch: Pack up some leftover stir-fry from yesterday and drizzle over a little extra soy sauce (make sure you have a vegan version). To brighten it up into a lunchtime salad, stir in fresh edamame beans and season lightly.
- Dinner: Pasta bake cooked with leeks, mushrooms, and a cheesy white sauce made with nutritional yeast. Sprinkle some toasted sunflower and pumpkin seeds on top, and serve with fresh spinach and tomatoes.

Thursday
- Breakfast: Prepare yourself some chia pudding the night before, and you'll have a tasty, high-protein breakfast to start the day. Add some sliced kiwi and star fruit in the morning so the fruit doesn't lose its crispness.
- Lunch: Moroccan couscous cooked in vegetable stock with diced eggplant, peppers, and tomatoes.
- Dinner: Cook up some wonderful fresh falafel, but save yourself a little hassle by serving alongside leftover couscous from lunchtime. Be sure to make a little extra falafel for lunch tomorrow!

Friday
- Breakfast: Slice up some fresh pineapple to keep you feeling zingy right through to the last day of the work week! Mix up some trail mix from your favorite nuts, seeds, and crackers to graze on throughout the morning.
- Lunch: Mix up some of yesterday's leftover falafel with shredded lettuce and sliced tomato. Serve in wraps with a little vegan mayo.
- Dinner: Friday night is pizza night! Cook up a tomato sauce with onions, garlic, and mushrooms. Puree the mixture with a stick blender and spread over ready-made pizza dough or flatbread bases (which

often contain only plant-based ingredients). You can then add your favorite pizza toppings – choose from sliced peppers, sliced vegan sausage, substitute mozzarella, pineapple chunks, jalapeno, mushrooms, and zucchini… The possibilities are endless.

Saturday
- Breakfast: Start your weekend off with a substantial fried breakfast. Cook up some beans in a tomato sauce to serve over hash browns or fried potatoes. Scramble some tofu with paprika, turmeric, and black onion seeds. Add some toast and garlic mushrooms, and you'll be set up for whatever adventures come your way!
- Lunch: After a big breakfast, you might not need a heavy lunch. Why not treat yourself to a fresh fruit smoothie whilst baking up a vegan cake? There are plenty of recipes to try online, and the weekend is a great time to relax with something fun in the kitchen.
- Dinner: Whether you're dining out or inviting friends round, a simple pasta dish can be a great option. Try roasting peaches and plums alongside tomatoes and peppers, and stir into high-quality pasta. Add some sun-dried tomato paste for a fresh and zingy flavor. A bowl of toasted sunflower and sesame seeds stirred through with sea salt and a good black pepper will make the perfect seasoning for your guests, and add a little protein punch.

Sunday
- Breakfast: Make yourself a good batch of granola today, and you can enjoy it into the following week. In a baking tray, stir together a couple of cups of oats, some chopped nuts and seeds, raisins, and diced dried apple, together with half a teaspoon of mixed spice. Add a couple of spoons of maple syrup, or your preferred sweetener, and mix well before putting into a hot oven. After ten minutes or so, take the tray out and mix everything again with a spatula. After another ten minutes in the oven, it should be starting to turn golden and ready to enjoy.
- Lunch: Put together a healthy green leaf salad for lunch and make a little extra to serve with tonight's evening meal.
- Dinner: Sunday meals are often a family event, so bake up a vegan lasagna that will please everyone. In one pan, cook up some orange lentils with passata, garlic and ginger. Add any chopped vegetables

which you might have left over from the week too. In another pan, make a white sauce using dairy-free spread, almond milk, and all-purpose flour. Once that has thickened, whisk in some silken tofu, seasoning, and nutritional yeast. Layer the lentil mixture and white sauce with egg-free lasagna sheets, and bake in a medium-high oven for around forty minutes. Serve with a green salad and a bottle of red wine!

CHAPTER 8

Eating Out

There is no denying that changing to a vegan diet will affect the way you order food when you're out – but that can be a good thing! It might be hard to imagine eating out and visiting the usual restaurants as a vegan, and it is certainly one of the big fears for those who are considering switching to a plant-based diet. Common worries include:

- Will there be any restaurants I can go to?
- Can I still eat fast food?
- Will my friends be offended or think I am being difficult if I insist on going to vegan places?
- How should I deal with invitations to dinner at other people's houses?
- How can I eat while traveling?

There are, of course, ways to deal with any and all of these situations. There are also ways in which your attitude shifts when eating a vegan diet. Things which used to seem appealing may no longer seem so attractive. People's attitudes and friendship groups can change, and restaurants are more accommodating than ever before. Here are 11 tips for dealing with the challenges of eating out while staying on a vegan diet:

1. Plan Ahead

It might sounds obvious, but forward planning really is the key to eating out and enjoying it as a vegan! Before you venture out for your first restaurant experience as a vegan, do some research and keep notes about places where you know you will be able to eat. Whether you keep an online file or make a physical list in a notebook, organize your findings into two groups:

2. Vegan Restaurants

With the interest in plant-based diets on the rise, it's no surprise that there seem to be new all-vegan eateries popping up all the time. But if you don't know where to look, they can be tricky to find. Sometimes that's because they are small businesses which don't have big marketing budgets, so they rely on word of mouth and their reputation amongst the vegan community in their area. Other times it's because a vegan-only restaurant becomes so popular that people forget it only offers vegan food!

The great thing about a vegan café or restaurant is, of course, that you will be able to choose anything from the menu without worrying about what it contains. This list will become your go-to reference point whenever you want to treat yourself to a meal out, to suggest a meeting place with other vegan friends, or for persuading non-vegan friends that plant-based food can be luxurious and exciting! It can be a nice feel-good experience to support a business with a vegan ethos too.

You will also find that specialist vegan restaurants often offer foods which are the latest internet trend, or which rely on unusual ingredients that are more difficult to obtain. So they can be great places to go to if you want to try jackfruit or seitan... or just an extravagant almond milk sundae!

3. Vegan-Friendly Restaurants

Whether or not an eatery is friendly to vegans isn't just about the menu – although that is, of course, important. The attitude of management, chefs, and waiting staff is also a really important factor in deciding whether or not a 'mainstream' restaurant is worth a visit. That is because some places may advertise several plant-based options but, if serving vegan customers isn't something they do often, you may find not all of them are available and your choice has been reduced to one – or none!

You should also be cautious of chain restaurants, or places which heavily rely on meat products, such as steakhouses. They may offer a vegan option, but if a restaurant isn't experienced in handling fresh ingredients or passionate about the taste of vegetables, the salad you're hoping will serve as a meal may turn out to be a plate of limp lettuce.

When you're checking out the restaurants local to you, have a browse of their menus online. Do they seem to feature vegetable-based options on the main menu or only as side dishes? Do they use symbols to designate foods which are completely free of animal products, or do you have to second-guess? Many restaurants now make their menus totally available online, so you could even print them off for future reference.

If you have an actual event or date night coming up on a particular day, call ahead and check what the menu options are likely to be that night. Not only will this give you a sense of whether there will be much for you and any vegan friends to choose from, but you will also get a sense of how friendly the place is to vegans in general. High-end restaurants and hotels may well offer to put something vegan together for you especially, even if their menu doesn't feature a single vegetarian dish! It's surprising where a bit of notice and a polite inquiry can get you.

4. Ask Around

If you're hiring a builder, or looking for someone to fix your computer, it's unlikely that you go with the first person whose name you find in the phone book or a Google search. Usually, we prefer to ask friends and family for recommendations, or at least check out some reviews online. Make sure you take the same approach when eating out if you want to be sure of the best possible experience.

Here are some tips for finding great vegan places to eat:
- Look on TripAdvisor
- Find vegan reviewers in your part of the world. Most countries or states have their own sites which collate information about vegan resources in that area. If you can't find specific vegan reviews, look for sites about vegetarian restaurants, as those often also offer vegan options.
- If you're in an area which doesn't seem to have many vegan offerings, try checking out your nearest Indian and Japanese restaurants. Many Indians are vegetarian, so they are likely to offer several plant-based options. Just ask them to hold off on the ghee! Many Japanese meals are also vegetarian or vegan. In fact, the Japanese approach to eating is thought to be one of the healthiest in the world!
- Extend your vegan social networks to find recommendations in your area. Join a local Facebook group for vegans or vegetarians, or use Twitter to identify vegan businesses near you. Check out your local wholefood shop too – they are often full of flyers and posters for local cafés and activities which are likely to be friendly to vegans and where you might meet other likeminded people.

5. Ordering in a Non-Vegan Restaurant

Sooner or later, you will probably find yourself unavoidably stuck in a situation where you need to order from a non-vegan menu. Maybe you'll be asked out with work colleagues at short notice so you don't have time to call ahead. Perhaps you will find yourself delayed while traveling in a strange town and need something to eat. Whatever the situation, there are a few key rules to getting through the experience without compromising on your diet or offending anyone around you.

Say what you want, but don't be one of 'those' customers.

Restaurants are usually really happy to help out vegan customers. This is particularly the case where things are cooked to order – just politely ask your server to see what the chef might be able to do for a vegan. Don't be demanding, but there is also no need to fall over yourself apologizing for any inconvenience caused. You are a paying customer, and the staff will want to help if they can.

6. Deal With Challenges From Those Around You Lightly

If you are eating out with non-vegan friends and family, you are likely to experience a range of comments and queries. Some people will be supportive and perhaps even show an interest. Others may raise an eyebrow and mind their own business. And sadly, a minority of people will always feel the need to seize the opportunity to probe a real-life vegan! Some people seem to expect that vegans will judge their own eating habits, so try not to be judgmental and perpetuate that stereotype. Don't feel that you have to lie about your reasons for going vegan if asked, though – just be honest without using language that will make others feel defensive and change the subject.

There will also be the odd few who will use even this sort of opportunity to show that veganism isn't necessary, or to make your choices appear silly. The best thing in a social situation is to give this sort of comment as little attention as possible without appearing rude or getting drawn into argument. You will never persuade this sort of person to change their mind, so just smile sweetly, give an honest reply, and move on… Sometimes humor can go a long way too!

7. Know How to Navigate a Non-Vegan Menu

If there isn't a single vegan dish on the menu and the kitchen won't be able to improvise, you will have to figure out something from the options which are available. If you are in a chain restaurant, you may well find that they are not able to simply make you a meat-free version of a dish. Many restaurants prepare courses in advance, and entire meals are often shipped to diners in plastic sealed packages which are then simply heated up and stirred through a little. Missing out on that sort of food is no great loss nutritionally, so sometimes it's best to just write the evening off, find something on the side menu, and plan to snack at home later!

8. Salads

The salad options are often the first port of call for those trying to navigate a regular menu whilst avoiding meat and dairy. However, it may not be as easy as it first seems. Many salad dressings feature honey or egg, and mayonnaise may feature too. If you can expect a decent dessert or plan to snack later, a dressing-free salad may suffice, but otherwise you may want to check out other parts of the menu.

9. Soups

Soup is of course often served as a starter, but most restaurants aren't too fussy about that. If there are no main vegan main courses, but a veggie soup features on the starter menu, why not ask if you can start with a salad and take the soup with some bread for your main course? It may also be possible to mix and match from other parts of the menu – perhaps some rice and veggies, with a bean chili or salad? Onion rings, soup, and greens? The options might not be quite right, but at least you will get a meal along with your friends!

10. Fries and Baked Potatoes

Fries are the easy option in any diner, café, or fast food joint when you simply need some carbs. They may not make a whole meal, but they can be substantial enough to stave off the hunger pangs! Asking for a portion of fries may not, however, feel appropriate in a classy restaurant. In that situation, you could ask whether the chef might prepare small jacket potatoes with salad, or potato croquettes with vegetables from one of the main courses.

11. Pre-Eat!

If you know you will be attending an event where there will not be any substantial vegan options available at all, there is only one sensible option… Have a good meal beforehand! That way you can graze at the side menu without your stomach rumbling. Whether or not you explain your reasons for not ordering properly is up to you – if you suspect it would cause offence or unwelcome enquiries, you could explain you are simply not very hungry. In most circumstances, however, it's best to simply be honest. Explain you are avoiding meat and dairy, and you knew there wouldn't be many options so you ate earlier, and don't mind at all. That should allow the conversation to move on without you needing to compromise yourself. If you're lucky, the next outing might be at a more vegan-friendly venue!

CHAPTER 9

Tips and Tricks to Help You Stay on a Vegan Diet

Deciding to switch to a vegan diet is one thing, but it can be quite another to stick with it. With so many common foods now off the menu, the pressure of social situations, nutritional requirements to balance, and new tastes to get used to, it's no wonder that many people struggle to stick with veganism in the long term.

The benefits of veganism, however, do not fade with time. The good reasons to go vegan – whether you are motivated by health or ethics, or both – will not change after a month, or a year, or on Christmas Day when the chocolates are being passed round! Many people, however, do stay vegan throughout all stages of their lives without a problem. Here are some points to remember if you'd like to stick with a plant-based diet in the long term. Why not write some of them out on sticky notes and put them on your fridge?

A Slip Is Not a Failure

Some vegans are passionate converts and slip instantly into full-time veganism. For most people, however, there will be some sort of transition period. Whether you decide to spend some time as a pescatarian (eating fish but not meat), vegetarian, or perhaps cutting out milk but not eggs, remember those are all valid steps on the path to veganism. Don't let anyone make you feel bad if you don't seem to be as perfectly vegan or ethical as they are – life is not a competition!

Most vegans will definitely experience slip-ups at some point too. Whether you have a weakness for something off-limits which occasionally seems to fall into your shopping bags, or have accidentally eaten something which you mistakenly assumed did not contain animal products, don't worry! This doesn't mean you have failed at your diet. Because there is also an ethical, animal rights aspect to the vegan way of life, people are particularly likely to feel guilty or ashamed when they fall off the wagon or find it hard to get the right sort of food while out and about. It's important that you try not to be too hard on yourself, though. Allow yourself to be imperfect, and you and the planet will benefit from your developing relationship with veganism.

Seek out Support

Veganism can feel isolating at times, especially if your friends or family don't seem to understand your reasons for making this dietary choice. If that's the case for you, why not try some of the tips from the eating out section to help you extend your networks? You could even start your own social media account to connect with like-minded people in your area and all around the world. Finding other vegans in real life and online can be inspiring, as it will expose you to new recipe and food ideas, but it can also be a source of advice and support in dealing with the fact that veganism can be regarded as an extreme diet.

Continue to Take Care of Your Health

Veganism is great for your health, but it is not a cure for every illness going! Just as with any other diet or major lifestyle change, you should consider what impact going vegan might have on your health and continue to monitor this as you continue with your new diet.

If you have any pre-existing digestive conditions, allergies, or other illnesses which require the exclusion of major foods, a recent experience of eating disorder, or any other serious condition, then you may wish to consult an expert in your area before proceeding. Try not to worry too much about doctors and other health practitioners criticizing your interest in veganism. They will have met plenty of vegans before, and will probably have noticed that they tend to have better health and to take an interest in positive lifestyle choices. You may also decide to seek out healthcare professionals who are likely to have more experience of veganism. If you are pregnant, breastfeeding, or raising young children on a vegan diet, you must take particular care to ensure that all of their nutritional requirements are met.

If you find yourself feeling very tired, or experiencing any other symptoms which are not usual for you, you should address that in the normal way. Some vegans can experience nutritional deficiencies as they adjust, and bloodwork or seeing a nutritionist might be helpful. But unusual symptoms can also be a sign of other illnesses, stress, or any other experience which non-vegans might have. Don't let anyone try and persuade you that your symptoms are your own fault for being vegan! Just take proper advice in whatever way you usually would.

Explore Broader Aspects of Veganism (but don't let your diet control your life!)

Many people first come to veganism for dietary reasons, and then come to learn about the ethical aspects as they become more conscious of the food which is being put into their bodies. This can lead to people taking an interest in animal rights, farming standards, and even political campaigning. It shouldn't mean you're a 'bad' vegan if you don't take an interest in these things, but it's always healthy to allow your mind to open up to new experiences. If you find you no longer feel like wearing leather now that you no longer consume beef or milk, then why not explore the available alternatives? Perhaps you will be part of a gradual change to a kinder society!

On the other hand, with a multi-faceted diet such as veganism, it can sometimes seem like everything becomes an 'issue'. Everything from breakfast to the clothes you wear and the people you associate with might come to be seen through vegan lenses! This is quite normal, as it is a big lifestyle change to make. Some people really enjoy the social and political aspects of veganism, and seek out work or business opportunities which allow them to incorporate their beliefs into every aspect of life. Of course, that is not the case for everyone, though! If you find that your vegan diet just becomes a normal part of life which is hardly worthy of comment, that's great too. In fact, it could set a great example to others considering a plant-based diet, who will be reassured to see that going vegan is not overly demanding.

Conclusion

Hopefully, this information will allow you to consider all the aspects of a vegan diet and decide whether it is right for you. There is no doubt that cutting out meat and dairy products helps many people feel better, both health-wise and in terms of their relationship to the environment. It's also true that going vegan is a big decision which should be carefully researched and planned for.

This guide should have deepened your insight into eating a plant-based diet, and provided useful information about nutritional requirements and practical issues. Whether or not you decide veganism is for you, it's certainly important to understand why more and more people are turning to fruits, vegetables, and grains over meat and dairy.